Table of Contents

Healthy Eating — A Detailed Guide for Beginners

The foods you eat have big effects on your health and quality of life.

Although eating healthy can be fairly simple, the rise in popular "diets" and dieting trends has caused confusion.

In fact, these trends often distract from the basic nutrition principles that are most important.

This is a detailed beginner's guide to healthy eating, based on the latest in nutrition science.

Why Should You Eat Healthy?

Research continues to link serious diseases to a poor diet.

For example, eating healthy can drastically reduce your chances of developing heart disease and cancer, the world's leading killers.

A good diet can improve all aspects of life, from brain function to physical performance. In fact, food affects all your cells and organs

If you participate in exercise or sports, there is no doubt that a healthy diet will help you perform better.

BOTTOM LINE:

From disease risk to brain function and physical performance, a healthy diet is vital for every aspect of life.

Calories and Energy Balance Explained

In recent years, the importance of calories has been pushed aside.

While calorie counting isn't always necessary, total calorie intake still plays a key role in weight control and health.

If you put in more calories than you burn, you will store them as new muscle or body fat. If you consume fewer calories than you burn every day, you will lose weight.

If you want to lose weight, you must create some form of calorie deficit.

In contrast, if you are trying to gain weight and increase muscle mass, then you need to eat more than your body burns.

BOTTOM LINE:

Calories and energy balance are important, regardless of the composition of your diet.

Understanding Macronutrients

The three macronutrients are carbohydrates (carbs), fats and protein.

These nutrients are needed in relatively large amounts. They provide calories and have various functions in your body.

Here are some common foods within each macronutrient group:

- Carbs: 4 calories per gram. All starchy foods like bread, pasta and potatoes. Also includes fruit, legumes, juice, sugar and some dairy products.

- Protein: 4 calories per gram. Main sources include meat and fish, dairy, eggs, legumes and vegetarian alternatives like tofu.

- Fats: 9 calories per gram. Main sources include nuts, seeds, oils, butter, cheese, oily fish and fatty meat.

How much of each macronutrient you should consume depends on your lifestyle and goals, as well as your personal preferences.

BOTTOM LINE:

Macronutrients are the three main nutrients needed in large amounts: carbs, fats and protein.

Understanding Micronutrients

Micronutrients are important vitamins and minerals that you require in smaller doses.

Some of the most common micronutrients you should know include:

- Magnesium: Plays a role in over 600 cellular processes, including energy production, nervous system function and muscle contraction.

- Potassium: This mineral is important for blood pressure control, fluid balance and the function of your muscles and nerves.

- Iron: Primarily known for carrying oxygen in the blood, iron also has many other benefits, including improved immune and brain function.

- Calcium: An important structural component of bones and teeth, and also a key mineral for your heart, muscles and nervous system.

- All vitamins: The vitamins, from vitamin A to K, play important roles in every organ and cell in your body.

All of the vitamins and minerals are "essential" nutrients, meaning that you must get them from the diet in order to survive.

The daily requirement of each micronutrient varies between individuals. If you eat a real food-based diet that includes plants and animals, then you should get all the micronutrients your body needs without taking a supplement.

BOTTOM LINE:

Micronutrients are important vitamins and minerals that play key roles in your cells and organs.

Eating Whole Foods is Important

You should aim to consume whole foods at least 80-90% of the time.

The term "whole foods" generally describes natural, unprocessed foods containing only one ingredient.

If the product looks like it was made in a factory, then it's probably not a whole food.

Whole foods tend to be nutrient-dense and have a lower energy density. This means that they have fewer calories and more nutrients per serving than processed foods.

In contrast, many processed foods have little nutritional value and are often referred to as "empty" calories. Eating them in large amounts is linked to obesity and other diseases.

BOTTOM LINE:

Basing your diet on whole foods is an extremely effective but simple strategy to improve health and lose weight.

Foods to Eat

Try to base your diet around these healthy food groups:

• Vegetables: These should play a fundamental role at most meals. They are low in calories yet full of important micronutrients and fiber.

• Fruits: A natural sweet treat, fruit provides micronutrients and antioxidants that can help improve health.

• Meat and fish: Meat and fish have been the major sources of protein throughout evolution. They are a staple in the human diet, although vegetarian and vegan diets have become popular as well.

• Nuts and seeds: These are one of the best fat sources available and also contain important micronutrients.

- Eggs: Considered one of the healthiest foods on the planet, whole eggs pack a powerful combination of protein, beneficial fats and micronutrients.

- Dairy: Dairy products such as natural yogurt and milk are convenient, low-cost sources of protein and calcium.

- Healthy starches: For those who aren't on a low-carb diet, whole food starchy foods like potatoes, quinoa and Ezekiel bread are healthy and nutritious.

- Beans and legumes: These are fantastic sources of fiber, protein and micronutrients.

- Beverages: Water should make up the majority of your fluid intake, along with drinks like coffee and tea.

- Herbs and spices: These are often very high in nutrients and beneficial plant compounds.

Foods to Avoid Most of the Time

By following the advice in this article, you will naturally reduce your intake of unhealthy foods.

No food needs to be eliminated forever, but some foods should be limited or saved for special occasions.

These include:

• Sugar-based products: Foods high in sugar, especially sugary drinks, are linked to obesity and type 2 diabetes.

• Trans fats: Also known as partially hydrogenated fats, trans fats have been linked to serious diseases, such as heart disease.

• Refined carbs: Foods that are high in refined carbs, such as white bread, are linked to overeating, obesity and metabolic disease.

• Vegetable oils: While many people believe these are healthy, vegetable oils can disrupt your body's omega 6-to-3 balance, which may cause problems.

• Processed low-fat products: Often disguised as healthy alternatives, low-fat products usually contain a lot of sugar to make them taste better.

BOTTOM LINE:

While no food is strictly off limits, overeating certain foods can increase disease risk and lead to weight gain.

Why Portion Control is Important

Your calorie intake is a key factor in weight control and health.

By controlling your portions, you are more likely to avoid consuming too many calories.

While whole foods are certainly a lot harder to overeat than processed foods, they can still be eaten in excess.

If you are overweight or trying to lose body fat, it's particularly important to monitor your portion size.

There are many simple strategies to control portion size.

For example, you can use smaller plates and take a smaller-than-average first serving, then wait 20 minutes before you return for more.

Another popular approach is measuring portion size with your hand.

An example meal would limit most people to 1 fist-sized portion of carbs, 1–2 palms of protein and 1–2 thumb-sized portions of healthy fats.

More calorie-dense foods such as cheese, nuts and fatty meats are healthy, but make sure you pay attention to portion sizes when you eat them.

BOTTOM LINE:

Be aware of portion sizes and your total food or calorie intake, especially if you are overweight or trying to lose fat.

How to Tailor Your Diet to Your Goals

First, assess your calorie needs based on factors like your activity levels and weight goals.

Quite simply, if you want to lose weight, you must eat less than you burn. If you want to gain weight, you should consume more calories than you burn.

Here is a calorie calculator that tells you how much you should eat, and here are 5 free websites and apps that help you track calories and nutrients.

If you dislike calorie counting, you can simply apply the rules discussed above, such as monitoring portion size and focusing on whole foods.

If you have a certain deficiency or are at risk of developing one, you may wish to tailor your diet to account for this. For instance, vegetarians or people who eliminate certain food groups are at greater risk of missing out on some nutrients.

In general, you should consume foods of various types and colors to ensure you get plenty of all the macro- and micronutrients.

While many debate whether low-carb or low-fat diets are best, the truth is that it depends on the individual.

Based on research, athletes and those looking to lose weight should consider increasing their protein intake. In addition, a lower-carb diet may work wonders for some individuals trying to lose weight or treat type 2 diabetes.

BOTTOM LINE:

Consider your total calorie intake and adjust your diet based on your own needs and goals.

How to Make Healthy Eating Sustainable

Here's a great rule to live by: If you can't see yourself on this diet in one, two or three years, then it's not right for you.

Far too often, people go on extreme diets they can't maintain, which means they never actually develop long-term, healthy eating habits.

There are some frightening weight gain statistics showing that most people regain all the weight they lost soon after attempting a weight loss diet.

As always, balance is key. Unless you have a specific disease or dietary requirement, no food needs to be off limits forever. By totally eliminating certain foods, you may actually increase cravings and decrease long-term success.

Basing 90% of your diet on whole foods and eating smaller portions will allow you to enjoy treats occasionally yet still achieve excellent health.

This is a far healthier approach than doing the opposite and eating 90% processed food and only 10% whole food like many people do.

BOTTOM LINE:

Create a healthy diet that you can enjoy and stick with for the long term. If you want unhealthy foods, save them for an occasional treat.

Consider These Supplements

As the name suggests, supplements are meant to be used in addition to a healthy diet.

Including plenty of nutrient-dense foods in your diet should help you reverse deficiencies and meet all your daily needs.

However, a few well-researched supplements have been shown to be helpful in some cases.

One example is vitamin D, which is naturally obtained from sunlight and foods like oily fish. Most people have low levels or are deficient.

Supplements like magnesium, zinc and omega-3s can provide additional benefits if you do not get enough of them from your diet.

Other supplements can be used to enhance sports performance. Creatine, whey protein and beta-alanine all have plenty of research supporting their use.

In a perfect world, your diet would be full of nutrient-dense foods with no need for supplements. However, this isn't always achievable in the real world.

If you are already making a constant effort to improve your diet, additional supplements can help take your health a step further.

BOTTOM LINE:

It is best to get most of your nutrients from whole foods. However, some supplements can be useful as well.

Combine Good Nutrition With Other Healthy Habits

Nutrition isn't the only thing that matters for optimal health.

Following a healthy diet and exercising can give you an even bigger health boost.

It is also crucial to get good sleep. Research shows that sleep is just as important as nutrition for disease risk and weight control.

Hydration and water intake are also important. Drink when you're thirsty and stay well hydrated all day.

Finally, try to minimize stress. Long-term stress is linked to many health problems.

BOTTOM LINE:

Optimal health goes way beyond just nutrition. Exercising, getting good sleep and minimizing stress is also crucial.

Take Home Message

The strategies outlined above will drastically improve your diet.

They will also boost your health, lower your disease risk and help you lose weight.